MY DAILY FOOD JOURNAL

BY:

SONYA A. BELL

FIRST PRINTING NOVEMBER 2024

ISBN : 978-1-7372949-9-3

PUBLISHED BY: BLU TOPAZ INC.

Photograph of Sonya A. Bell
by Tracy Horn

Dedicated to :

the families navigating the unique challenges of ADHD and autism, and to the children whose brilliance radiates with the power of nourishing foods.
As well as to the individual ready for change; may this journal be your guide to healing, connection, and hope.

BEYOND Radiant HEALTH COACHING

THIS JOURNAL BELONGS TO:

MY FOOD JOURNAL

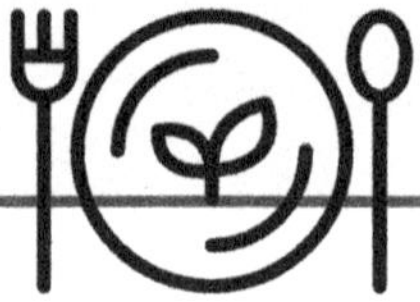

MEAL	DATE_____	DATE_____	DATE_____
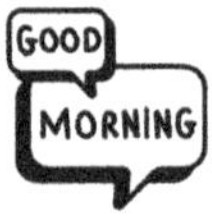 BREAKFAST (FOOD & BEVERAGE)			
SNACKS			
 LUNCH (FOOD & BEVERAGE)			
SNACKS			
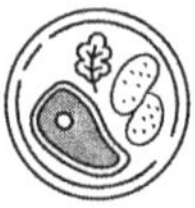 DINNER (FOOD & BEVERAGE)			
BM (HOW MANY BOWEL MOVEMENTS TODAY AND WAS IT HARD OR SOFT, WITH OR WITHOUT STRAINING?			
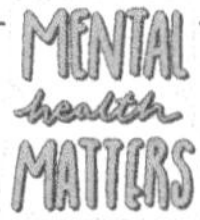	Behavior	Behavior	Behavior

MY FOOD JOURNAL

MEAL	DATE_____	DATE_____	DATE_____
BREAKFAST (FOOD & BEVERAGE)			
SNACKS			
LUNCH (FOOD & BEVERAGE)			
SNACKS			
DINNER (FOOD & BEVERAGE)			
BM (HOW MANY BOWEL MOVEMENTS TODAY AND WAS IT HARD OR SOFT, WITH OR WITHOUT STRAINING?			

Behavior Behavior Behavior

MY FOOD JOURNAL

MEAL	DATE_____	DATE_____	DATE_____
GOOD MORNING BREAKFAST (FOOD & BEVERAGE)			
SNACKS			
LUNCH TIME LUNCH (FOOD & BEVERAGE)			
SNACKS			
DINNER (FOOD & BEVERAGE)			
BM (HOW MANY BOWEL MOVEMENTS TODAY AND WAS IT HARD OR SOFT, WITH OR WITHOUT STRAINING?			
MENTAL health MATTERS	Behavior	Behavior	Behavior

MY FOOD JOURNAL

MEAL	DATE_____	DATE_____	DATE_____
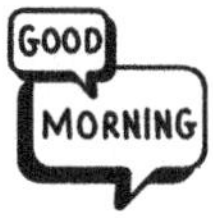 BREAKFAST (FOOD & BEVERAGE)			
SNACKS			
 LUNCH (FOOD & BEVERAGE)			
SNACKS			
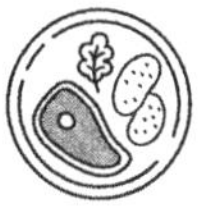 DINNER (FOOD & BEVERAGE)			
BM (HOW MANY BOWEL MOVEMENTS TODAY AND WAS IT HARD OR SOFT, WITH OR WITHOUT STRAINING?			

MENTAL health MATTERS

	Behavior	Behavior	Behavior

MY FOOD JOURNAL

MEAL	DATE_____	DATE_____	DATE_____
GOOD MORNING BREAKFAST (FOOD & BEVERAGE)			
SNACKS			
LUNCH TIME LUNCH (FOOD & BEVERAGE)			
SNACKS			
DINNER (FOOD & BEVERAGE)			
BM (HOW MANY BOWEL MOVEMENTS TODAY AND WAS IT HARD OR SOFT, WITH OR WITHOUT STRAINING?			
MENTAL health MATTERS	Behavior	Behavior	Behavior

MY FOOD JOURNAL

MEAL	DATE_____	DATE_____	DATE_____
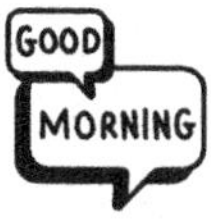 BREAKFAST (FOOD & BEVERAGE)			
SNACKS			
 LUNCH (FOOD & BEVERAGE)			
SNACKS			
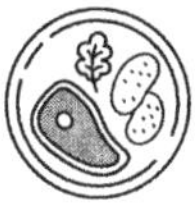 DINNER (FOOD & BEVERAGE)			
BM (HOW MANY BOWEL MOVEMENTS TODAY AND WAS IT HARD OR SOFT, WITH OR WITHOUT STRAINING?			
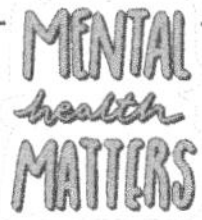	Behavior	Behavior	Behavior

MY FOOD JOURNAL

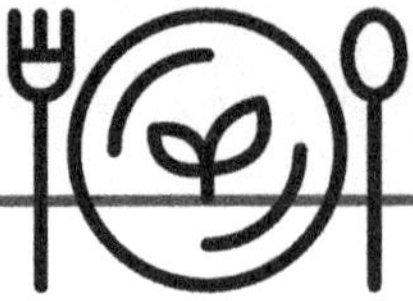

MEAL	DATE_____	DATE_____	DATE_____
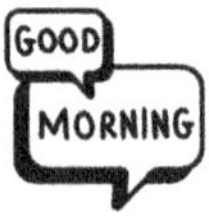 BREAKFAST (FOOD & BEVERAGE)			
SNACKS			
 LUNCH (FOOD & BEVERAGE)			
SNACKS			
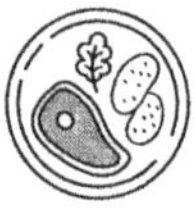 DINNER (FOOD & BEVERAGE)			
BM (HOW MANY BOWEL MOVEMENTS TODAY AND WAS IT HARD OR SOFT, WITH OR WITHOUT STRAINING?			
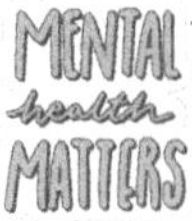	Behavior	Behavior	Behavior

MY FOOD JOURNAL

MEAL	DATE_____	DATE_____	DATE_____
GOOD MORNING BREAKFAST (FOOD & BEVERAGE)			
SNACKS			
LUNCH TIME LUNCH (FOOD & BEVERAGE)			
SNACKS			
DINNER (FOOD & BEVERAGE)			
BM (HOW MANY BOWEL MOVEMENTS TODAY AND WAS IT HARD OR SOFT, WITH OR WITHOUT STRAINING?			
MENTAL health MATTERS	Behavior	Behavior	Behavior

MY FOOD JOURNAL

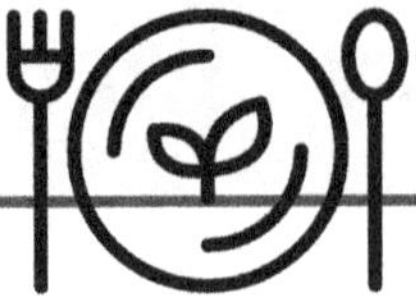

MEAL	DATE_____	DATE_____	DATE_____
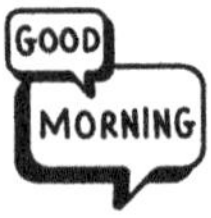 BREAKFAST (FOOD & BEVERAGE)			
SNACKS			
 LUNCH (FOOD & BEVERAGE)			
SNACKS			
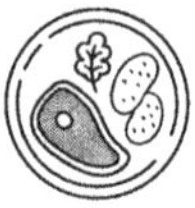 DINNER (FOOD & BEVERAGE)			
BM (HOW MANY BOWEL MOVEMENTS TODAY AND WAS IT HARD OR SOFT, WITH OR WITHOUT STRAINING?			

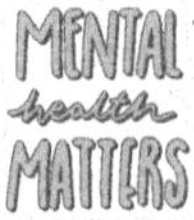

Behavior

Behavior

Behavior

MY FOOD JOURNAL

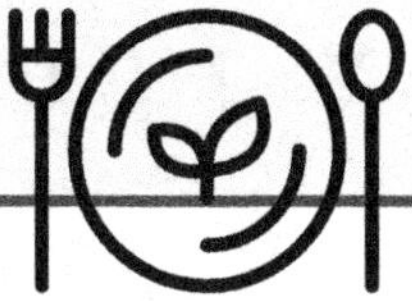

MEAL	DATE_____	DATE_____	DATE_____
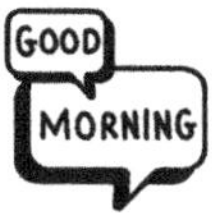 BREAKFAST (FOOD & BEVERAGE)			
SNACKS			
 LUNCH (FOOD & BEVERAGE)			
SNACKS			
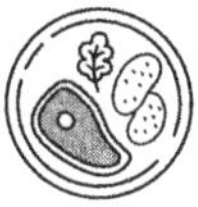 DINNER (FOOD & BEVERAGE)			
BM (HOW MANY BOWEL MOVEMENTS TODAY AND WAS IT HARD OR SOFT, WITH OR WITHOUT STRAINING?			

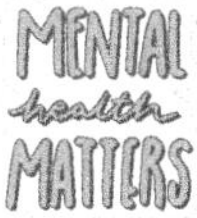

Behavior	Behavior	Behavior

MY FOOD JOURNAL

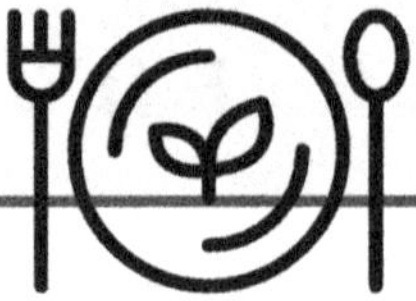

MEAL	DATE_____	DATE_____	DATE_____
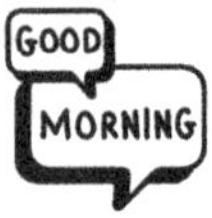 BREAKFAST (FOOD & BEVERAGE)			
SNACKS			
 LUNCH (FOOD & BEVERAGE)			
SNACKS			
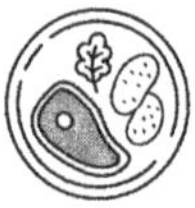 DINNER (FOOD & BEVERAGE)			
BM (HOW MANY BOWEL MOVEMENTS TODAY AND WAS IT HARD OR SOFT, WITH OR WITHOUT STRAINING?			
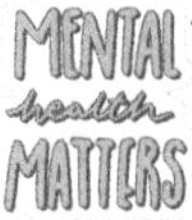	Behavior	Behavior	Behavior

MY FOOD JOURNAL

MEAL	DATE_____	DATE_____	DATE_____
BREAKFAST (FOOD & BEVERAGE)			
SNACKS			
LUNCH (FOOD & BEVERAGE)			
SNACKS			
DINNER (FOOD & BEVERAGE)			
BM (HOW MANY BOWEL MOVEMENTS TODAY AND WAS IT HARD OR SOFT, WITH OR WITHOUT STRAINING?			
MENTAL health MATTERS	Behavior	Behavior	Behavior

MY FOOD JOURNAL

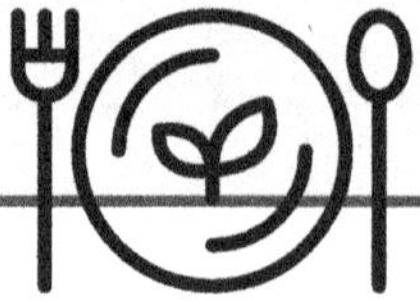

MEAL	DATE_____	DATE_____	DATE_____
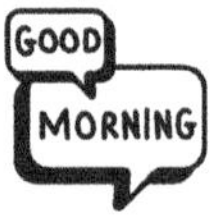 BREAKFAST (FOOD & BEVERAGE)			
SNACKS			
 LUNCH (FOOD & BEVERAGE)			
SNACKS			
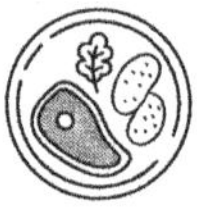 DINNER (FOOD & BEVERAGE)			
BM (HOW MANY BOWEL MOVEMENTS TODAY AND WAS IT HARD OR SOFT, WITH OR WITHOUT STRAINING?			
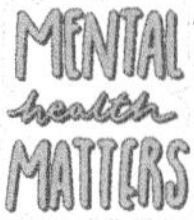	Behavior	Behavior	Behavior

MY FOOD JOURNAL

MEAL	DATE_____	DATE_____	DATE_____
GOOD MORNING BREAKFAST (FOOD & BEVERAGE)			
SNACKS			
LUNCH TIME LUNCH (FOOD & BEVERAGE)			
SNACKS			
DINNER (FOOD & BEVERAGE)			
BM (HOW MANY BOWEL MOVEMENTS TODAY AND WAS IT HARD OR SOFT, WITH OR WITHOUT STRAINING?			
MENTAL health MATTERS	Behavior	Behavior	Behavior

MY FOOD JOURNAL

MEAL	DATE_____	DATE_____	DATE_____
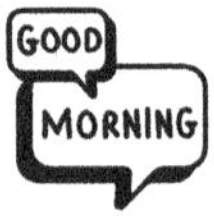 BREAKFAST (FOOD & BEVERAGE)			
SNACKS			
 LUNCH (FOOD & BEVERAGE)			
SNACKS			
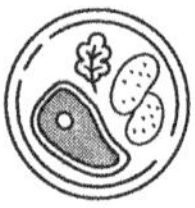 DINNER (FOOD & BEVERAGE)			
BM (HOW MANY BOWEL MOVEMENTS TODAY AND WAS IT HARD OR SOFT, WITH OR WITHOUT STRAINING?			
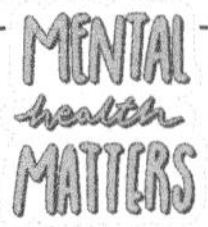	Behavior	Behavior	Behavior

MY FOOD JOURNAL

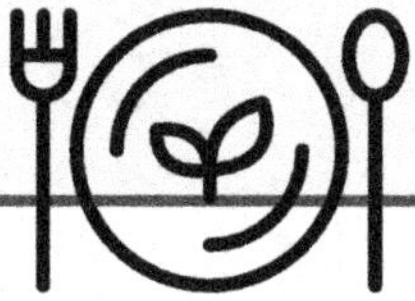

MEAL	DATE_____	DATE_____	DATE_____
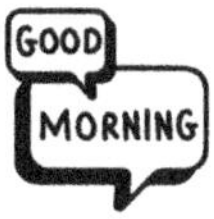 BREAKFAST (FOOD & BEVERAGE)			
SNACKS			
 LUNCH (FOOD & BEVERAGE)			
SNACKS			
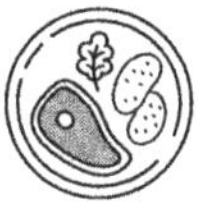 DINNER (FOOD & BEVERAGE)			
BM (HOW MANY BOWEL MOVEMENTS TODAY AND WAS IT HARD OR SOFT, WITH OR WITHOUT STRAINING?			

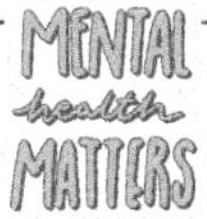

Behavior

Behavior

Behavior

MY FOOD JOURNAL

MEAL	DATE_____	DATE_____	DATE_____
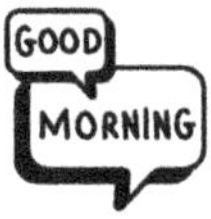 BREAKFAST (FOOD & BEVERAGE)			
SNACKS			
 LUNCH (FOOD & BEVERAGE)			
SNACKS			
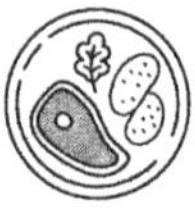 DINNER (FOOD & BEVERAGE)			
BM (HOW MANY BOWEL MOVEMENTS TODAY AND WAS IT HARD OR SOFT, WITH OR WITHOUT STRAINING?			
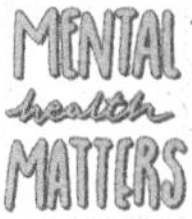	Behavior	Behavior	Behavior

MY FOOD JOURNAL

MEAL	DATE_____	DATE_____	DATE_____
GOOD MORNING BREAKFAST (FOOD & BEVERAGE)			
SNACKS			
LUNCH TIME LUNCH (FOOD & BEVERAGE)			
SNACKS			
DINNER (FOOD & BEVERAGE)			
BM (HOW MANY BOWEL MOVEMENTS TODAY AND WAS IT HARD OR SOFT, WITH OR WITHOUT STRAINING?			

MENTAL health MATTERS

Behavior	Behavior	Behavior

MY FOOD JOURNAL

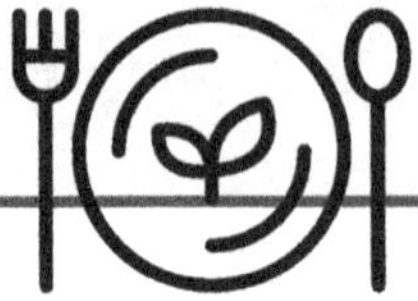

MEAL	DATE_____	DATE_____	DATE_____
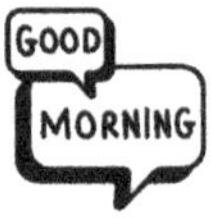 BREAKFAST (FOOD & BEVERAGE)			
SNACKS			
 LUNCH (FOOD & BEVERAGE)			
SNACKS			
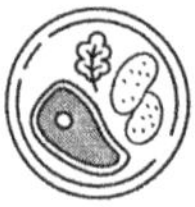 DINNER (FOOD & BEVERAGE)			
BM (HOW MANY BOWEL MOVEMENTS TODAY AND WAS IT HARD OR SOFT, WITH OR WITHOUT STRAINING?			
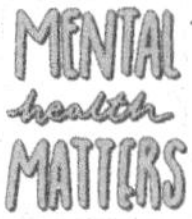	Behavior	Behavior	Behavior

MY FOOD JOURNAL

MEAL	DATE_____	DATE_____	DATE_____
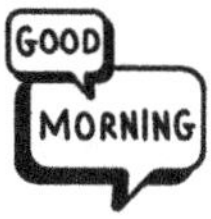 BREAKFAST (FOOD & BEVERAGE)			
SNACKS			
 LUNCH (FOOD & BEVERAGE)			
SNACKS			
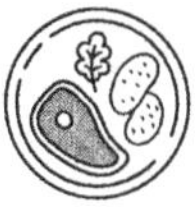 DINNER (FOOD & BEVERAGE)			
BM (HOW MANY BOWEL MOVEMENTS TODAY AND WAS IT HARD OR SOFT, WITH OR WITHOUT STRAINING?			

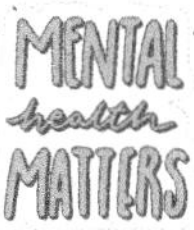

Behavior

Behavior

Behavior

MY FOOD JOURNAL

MEAL	DATE_____	DATE_____	DATE_____
GOOD MORNING BREAKFAST (FOOD & BEVERAGE)			
SNACKS			
LUNCH TIME LUNCH (FOOD & BEVERAGE)			
SNACKS			
DINNER (FOOD & BEVERAGE)			
BM (HOW MANY BOWEL MOVEMENTS TODAY AND WAS IT HARD OR SOFT, WITH OR WITHOUT STRAINING?			
MENTAL health MATTERS	Behavior	Behavior	Behavior

MY FOOD JOURNAL

MEAL	DATE_____	DATE_____	DATE_____
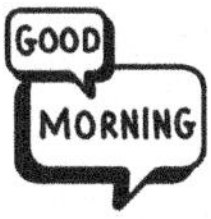 BREAKFAST (FOOD & BEVERAGE)			
SNACKS			
 LUNCH (FOOD & BEVERAGE)			
SNACKS			
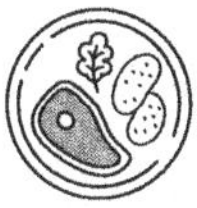 DINNER (FOOD & BEVERAGE)			
BM (HOW MANY BOWEL MOVEMENTS TODAY AND WAS IT HARD OR SOFT, WITH OR WITHOUT STRAINING?			

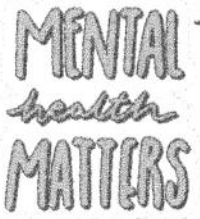

	Behavior	Behavior	Behavior

MY FOOD JOURNAL

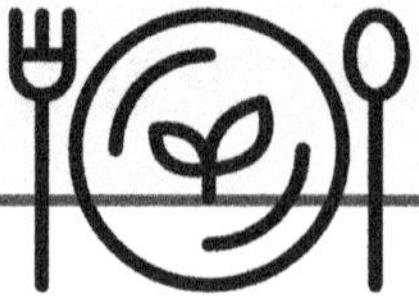

MEAL	DATE_____	DATE_____	DATE_____
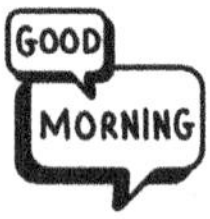 BREAKFAST (FOOD & BEVERAGE)			
SNACKS			
 LUNCH (FOOD & BEVERAGE)			
SNACKS			
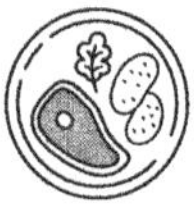 DINNER (FOOD & BEVERAGE)			
BM (HOW MANY BOWEL MOVEMENTS TODAY AND WAS IT HARD OR SOFT, WITH OR WITHOUT STRAINING?			
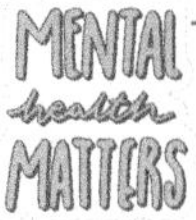	Behavior	Behavior	Behavior

MY FOOD JOURNAL

MEAL	DATE_____	DATE_____	DATE_____
BREAKFAST (FOOD & BEVERAGE)			
SNACKS			
LUNCH (FOOD & BEVERAGE)			
SNACKS			
DINNER (FOOD & BEVERAGE)			
BM (HOW MANY BOWEL MOVEMENTS TODAY AND WAS IT HARD OR SOFT, WITH OR WITHOUT STRAINING?			
	Behavior	Behavior	Behavior

MY FOOD JOURNAL

MEAL	DATE_____	DATE_____	DATE_____
BREAKFAST (FOOD & BEVERAGE)			
SNACKS			
LUNCH (FOOD & BEVERAGE)			
SNACKS			
DINNER (FOOD & BEVERAGE)			
BM (HOW MANY BOWEL MOVEMENTS TODAY AND WAS IT HARD OR SOFT, WITH OR WITHOUT STRAINING?			
	Behavior	Behavior	Behavior

MY FOOD JOURNAL

MEAL	DATE_____	DATE_____	DATE_____
BREAKFAST (FOOD & BEVERAGE)			
SNACKS			
LUNCH (FOOD & BEVERAGE)			
SNACKS			
DINNER (FOOD & BEVERAGE)			
BM (HOW MANY BOWEL MOVEMENTS TODAY AND WAS IT HARD OR SOFT, WITH OR WITHOUT STRAINING?			

Behavior

Behavior

Behavior

MY FOOD JOURNAL

MEAL	DATE_____	DATE_____	DATE_____
GOOD MORNING BREAKFAST (FOOD & BEVERAGE)			
SNACKS			
LUNCH TIME LUNCH (FOOD & BEVERAGE)			
SNACKS			
DINNER (FOOD & BEVERAGE)			
BM (HOW MANY BOWEL MOVEMENTS TODAY AND WAS IT HARD OR SOFT, WITH OR WITHOUT STRAINING?			
MENTAL health MATTERS	Behavior	Behavior	Behavior

MY FOOD JOURNAL

MEAL	DATE_____	DATE_____	DATE_____
GOOD MORNING BREAKFAST (FOOD & BEVERAGE)			
SNACKS			
LUNCH TIME LUNCH (FOOD & BEVERAGE)			
SNACKS			
DINNER (FOOD & BEVERAGE)			
BM (HOW MANY BOWEL MOVEMENTS TODAY AND WAS IT HARD OR SOFT, WITH OR WITHOUT STRAINING?			
MENTAL health MATTERS	Behavior	Behavior	Behavior

MY FOOD JOURNAL

MEAL	DATE_____	DATE_____	DATE_____
BREAKFAST (FOOD & BEVERAGE)			
SNACKS			
LUNCH (FOOD & BEVERAGE)			
SNACKS			
DINNER (FOOD & BEVERAGE)			
BM (HOW MANY BOWEL MOVEMENTS TODAY AND WAS IT HARD OR SOFT, WITH OR WITHOUT STRAINING?			
	Behavior	Behavior	Behavior

MY FOOD JOURNAL

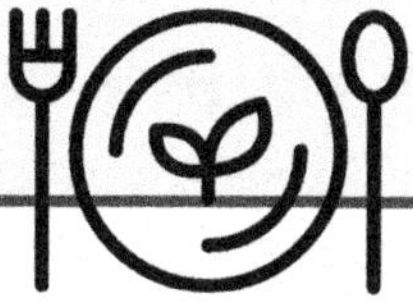

MEAL	DATE_____	DATE_____	DATE_____
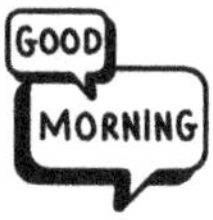 BREAKFAST (FOOD & BEVERAGE)			
SNACKS			
 LUNCH (FOOD & BEVERAGE)			
SNACKS			
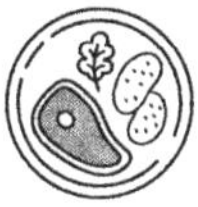 DINNER (FOOD & BEVERAGE)			
BM (HOW MANY BOWEL MOVEMENTS TODAY AND WAS IT HARD OR SOFT, WITH OR WITHOUT STRAINING?			

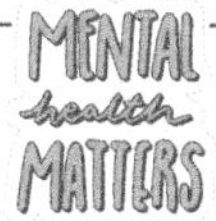

Behavior | Behavior | Behavior

MY FOOD JOURNAL

MEAL	DATE_____	DATE_____	DATE_____
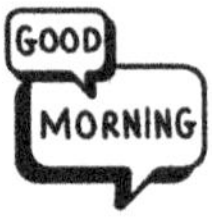 BREAKFAST (FOOD & BEVERAGE)			
SNACKS			
 LUNCH (FOOD & BEVERAGE)			
SNACKS			
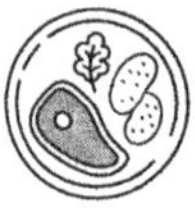 DINNER (FOOD & BEVERAGE)			
BM (HOW MANY BOWEL MOVEMENTS TODAY AND WAS IT HARD OR SOFT, WITH OR WITHOUT STRAINING?			
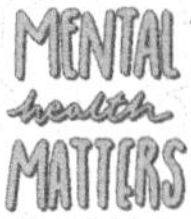	Behavior	Behavior	Behavior

MY FOOD JOURNAL

MEAL	DATE_____	DATE_____	DATE_____
BREAKFAST (FOOD & BEVERAGE)			
SNACKS			
LUNCH (FOOD & BEVERAGE)			
SNACKS			
DINNER (FOOD & BEVERAGE)			
BM (HOW MANY BOWEL MOVEMENTS TODAY AND WAS IT HARD OR SOFT, WITH OR WITHOUT STRAINING?			

Behavior	Behavior	Behavior

MY FOOD JOURNAL

MEAL	DATE_____	DATE_____	DATE_____
BREAKFAST (FOOD & BEVERAGE)			
SNACKS			
LUNCH (FOOD & BEVERAGE)			
SNACKS			
DINNER (FOOD & BEVERAGE)			
BM (HOW MANY BOWEL MOVEMENTS TODAY AND WAS IT HARD OR SOFT, WITH OR WITHOUT STRAINING?			
	Behavior	Behavior	Behavior

MY FOOD JOURNAL

MEAL	DATE_____	DATE_____	DATE_____
GOOD MORNING BREAKFAST (FOOD & BEVERAGE)			
SNACKS			
LUNCH TIME LUNCH (FOOD & BEVERAGE)			
SNACKS			
DINNER (FOOD & BEVERAGE)			
BM (HOW MANY BOWEL MOVEMENTS TODAY AND WAS IT HARD OR SOFT, WITH OR WITHOUT STRAINING?			
MENTAL health MATTERS	Behavior	Behavior	Behavior

MY FOOD JOURNAL

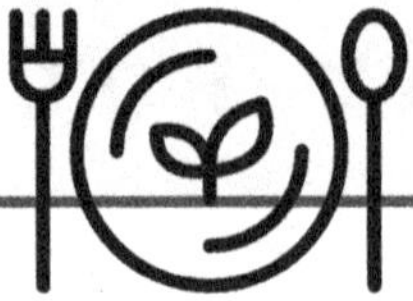

MEAL	DATE_____	DATE_____	DATE_____
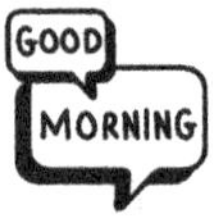 BREAKFAST (FOOD & BEVERAGE)			
SNACKS			
 LUNCH (FOOD & BEVERAGE)			
SNACKS			
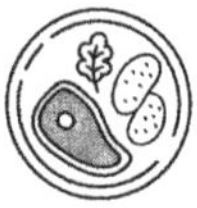 DINNER (FOOD & BEVERAGE)			
BM (HOW MANY BOWEL MOVEMENTS TODAY AND WAS IT HARD OR SOFT, WITH OR WITHOUT STRAINING?			
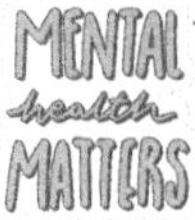	Behavior	Behavior	Behavior

MY FOOD JOURNAL

MEAL	DATE_____	DATE_____	DATE_____
BREAKFAST (FOOD & BEVERAGE)			
SNACKS			
LUNCH (FOOD & BEVERAGE)			
SNACKS			
DINNER (FOOD & BEVERAGE)			
BM (HOW MANY BOWEL MOVEMENTS TODAY AND WAS IT HARD OR SOFT, WITH OR WITHOUT STRAINING?			

Behavior	Behavior	Behavior

MY FOOD JOURNAL

MEAL	DATE_____	DATE_____	DATE_____
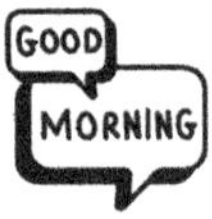 BREAKFAST (FOOD & BEVERAGE)			
SNACKS			
 LUNCH (FOOD & BEVERAGE)			
SNACKS			
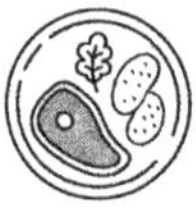 DINNER (FOOD & BEVERAGE)			
BM (HOW MANY BOWEL MOVEMENTS TODAY AND WAS IT HARD OR SOFT, WITH OR WITHOUT STRAINING?			
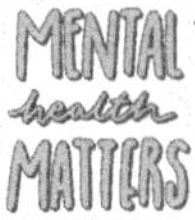	Behavior	Behavior	Behavior

MY FOOD JOURNAL

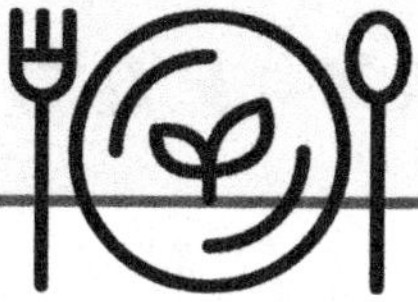

MEAL	DATE_____	DATE_____	DATE_____
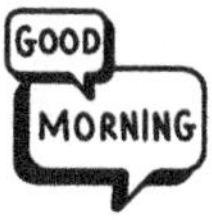 BREAKFAST (FOOD & BEVERAGE)			
SNACKS			
 LUNCH (FOOD & BEVERAGE)			
SNACKS			
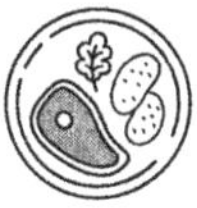 DINNER (FOOD & BEVERAGE)			
BM (HOW MANY BOWEL MOVEMENTS TODAY AND WAS IT HARD OR SOFT, WITH OR WITHOUT STRAINING?			

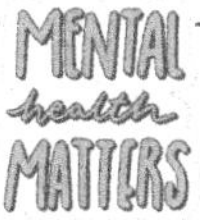

Behavior

Behavior

Behavior

MY FOOD JOURNAL

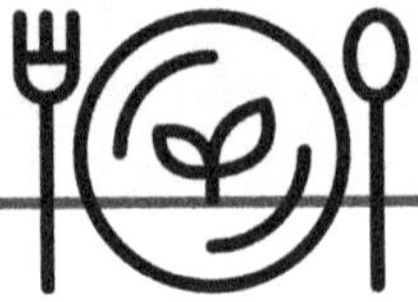

MEAL	DATE_____	DATE_____	DATE_____
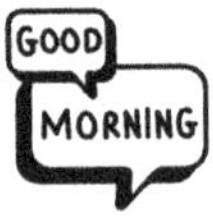 BREAKFAST (FOOD & BEVERAGE)			
SNACKS			
 LUNCH (FOOD & BEVERAGE)			
SNACKS			
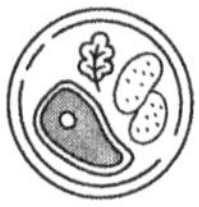 DINNER (FOOD & BEVERAGE)			
BM (HOW MANY BOWEL MOVEMENTS TODAY AND WAS IT HARD OR SOFT, WITH OR WITHOUT STRAINING?			

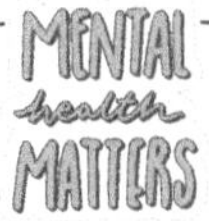

Behavior

Behavior

Behavior

MY FOOD JOURNAL

MEAL	DATE_____	DATE_____	DATE_____
BREAKFAST (FOOD & BEVERAGE)			
SNACKS			
LUNCH (FOOD & BEVERAGE)			
SNACKS			
DINNER (FOOD & BEVERAGE)			
BM (HOW MANY BOWEL MOVEMENTS TODAY AND WAS IT HARD OR SOFT, WITH OR WITHOUT STRAINING?			

MENTAL health MATTERS

Behavior

Behavior

Behavior

MY FOOD JOURNAL

MEAL	DATE_____	DATE_____	DATE_____
GOOD MORNING BREAKFAST (FOOD & BEVERAGE)			
SNACKS			
LUNCH TIME LUNCH (FOOD & BEVERAGE)			
SNACKS			
DINNER (FOOD & BEVERAGE)			
BM (HOW MANY BOWEL MOVEMENTS TODAY AND WAS IT HARD OR SOFT, WITH OR WITHOUT STRAINING?			
MENTAL health MATTERS	Behavior	Behavior	Behavior

MY FOOD JOURNAL

MEAL	DATE_____	DATE_____	DATE_____
BREAKFAST (FOOD & BEVERAGE)			
SNACKS			
LUNCH (FOOD & BEVERAGE)			
SNACKS			
DINNER (FOOD & BEVERAGE)			
BM (HOW MANY BOWEL MOVEMENTS TODAY AND WAS IT HARD OR SOFT, WITH OR WITHOUT STRAINING?			
	Behavior	Behavior	Behavior

MY FOOD JOURNAL

MEAL	DATE_____	DATE_____	DATE_____
GOOD MORNING BREAKFAST (FOOD & BEVERAGE)			
SNACKS			
LUNCH TIME LUNCH (FOOD & BEVERAGE)			
SNACKS			
DINNER (FOOD & BEVERAGE)			
BM (HOW MANY BOWEL MOVEMENTS TODAY AND WAS IT HARD OR SOFT, WITH OR WITHOUT STRAINING?			
MENTAL health MATTERS	Behavior	Behavior	Behavior

MY FOOD JOURNAL

MEAL	DATE_____	DATE_____	DATE_____
GOOD MORNING BREAKFAST (FOOD & BEVERAGE)			
SNACKS			
LUNCH TIME LUNCH (FOOD & BEVERAGE)			
SNACKS			
DINNER (FOOD & BEVERAGE)			
BM (HOW MANY BOWEL MOVEMENTS TODAY AND WAS IT HARD OR SOFT, WITH OR WITHOUT STRAINING?			
MENTAL health MATTERS	Behavior	Behavior	Behavior

MY FOOD JOURNAL

MEAL	DATE_____	DATE_____	DATE_____
GOOD MORNING BREAKFAST (FOOD & BEVERAGE)			
SNACKS			
LUNCH TIME LUNCH (FOOD & BEVERAGE)			
SNACKS			
DINNER (FOOD & BEVERAGE)			
BM (HOW MANY BOWEL MOVEMENTS TODAY AND WAS IT HARD OR SOFT, WITH OR WITHOUT STRAINING?			
MENTAL health MATTERS	Behavior	Behavior	Behavior

MY FOOD JOURNAL

MEAL	DATE_____	DATE_____	DATE_____
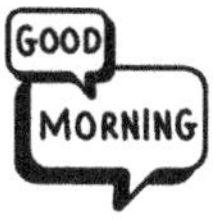 BREAKFAST (FOOD & BEVERAGE)			
SNACKS			
 LUNCH (FOOD & BEVERAGE)			
SNACKS			
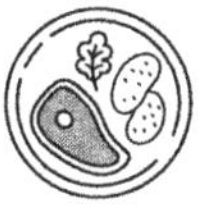 DINNER (FOOD & BEVERAGE)			
BM (HOW MANY BOWEL MOVEMENTS TODAY AND WAS IT HARD OR SOFT, WITH OR WITHOUT STRAINING?			
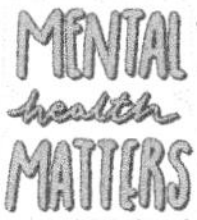	Behavior	Behavior	Behavior

MY FOOD JOURNAL

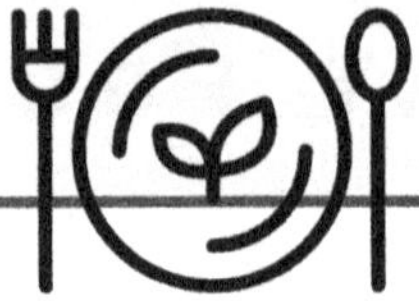

MEAL	DATE_____	DATE_____	DATE_____
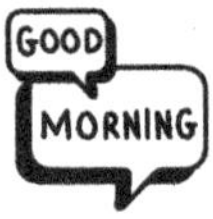 BREAKFAST (FOOD & BEVERAGE)			
SNACKS			
 LUNCH (FOOD & BEVERAGE)			
SNACKS			
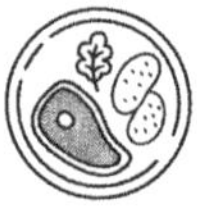 DINNER (FOOD & BEVERAGE)			
BM (HOW MANY BOWEL MOVEMENTS TODAY AND WAS IT HARD OR SOFT, WITH OR WITHOUT STRAINING?			
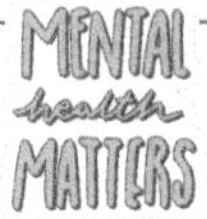	Behavior	Behavior	Behavior

MY FOOD JOURNAL

MEAL	DATE_____	DATE_____	DATE_____
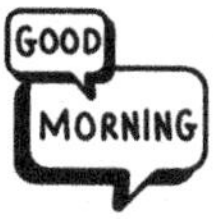 BREAKFAST (FOOD & BEVERAGE)			
SNACKS			
 LUNCH (FOOD & BEVERAGE)			
SNACKS			
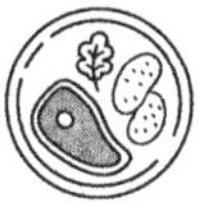 DINNER (FOOD & BEVERAGE)			
BM (HOW MANY BOWEL MOVEMENTS TODAY AND WAS IT HARD OR SOFT, WITH OR WITHOUT STRAINING?			

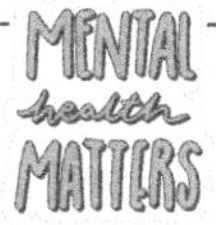

Behavior

Behavior

Behavior

MY FOOD JOURNAL

MEAL	DATE_____	DATE_____	DATE_____
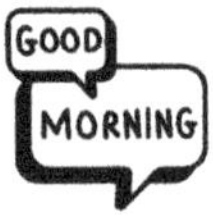 BREAKFAST (FOOD & BEVERAGE)			
SNACKS			
 LUNCH (FOOD & BEVERAGE)			
SNACKS			
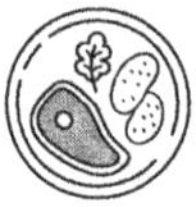 DINNER (FOOD & BEVERAGE)			
BM (HOW MANY BOWEL MOVEMENTS TODAY AND WAS IT HARD OR SOFT, WITH OR WITHOUT STRAINING?			
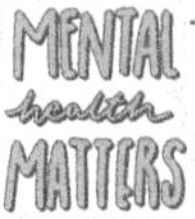	Behavior	Behavior	Behavior

MY FOOD JOURNAL

MEAL	DATE_____	DATE_____	DATE_____
GOOD MORNING BREAKFAST (FOOD & BEVERAGE)			
SNACKS			
LUNCH TIME LUNCH (FOOD & BEVERAGE)			
SNACKS			
DINNER (FOOD & BEVERAGE)			
BM (HOW MANY BOWEL MOVEMENTS TODAY AND WAS IT HARD OR SOFT, WITH OR WITHOUT STRAINING?			
MENTAL health MATTERS	Behavior	Behavior	Behavior

MY FOOD JOURNAL

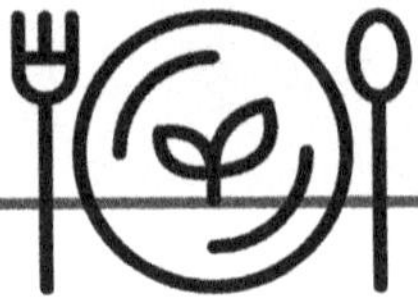

MEAL	DATE_____	DATE_____	DATE_____
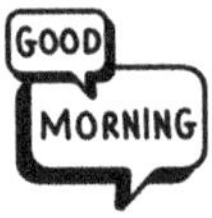 BREAKFAST (FOOD & BEVERAGE)			
SNACKS			
 LUNCH (FOOD & BEVERAGE)			
SNACKS			
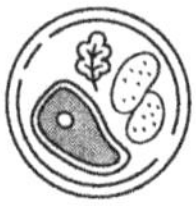 DINNER (FOOD & BEVERAGE)			
BM (HOW MANY BOWEL MOVEMENTS TODAY AND WAS IT HARD OR SOFT, WITH OR WITHOUT STRAINING?			
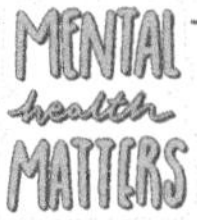	Behavior	Behavior	Behavior

MY FOOD JOURNAL

MEAL	DATE_____	DATE_____	DATE_____
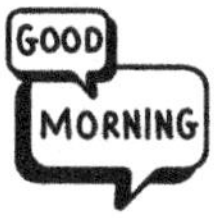 BREAKFAST (FOOD & BEVERAGE)			
SNACKS			
 LUNCH (FOOD & BEVERAGE)			
SNACKS			
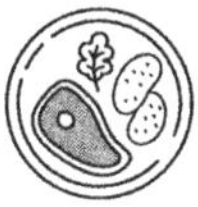 DINNER (FOOD & BEVERAGE)			
BM (HOW MANY BOWEL MOVEMENTS TODAY AND WAS IT HARD OR SOFT, WITH OR WITHOUT STRAINING?			
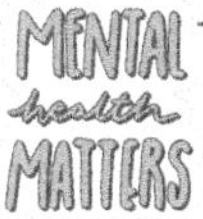	Behavior	Behavior	Behavior

MY FOOD JOURNAL

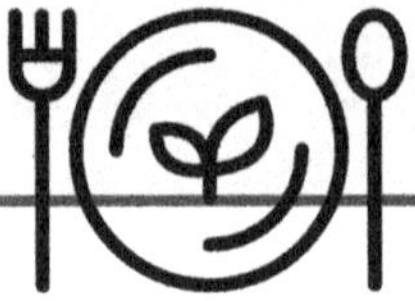

MEAL	DATE_____	DATE_____	DATE_____
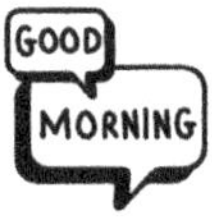 BREAKFAST (FOOD & BEVERAGE)			
SNACKS			
 LUNCH (FOOD & BEVERAGE)			
SNACKS			
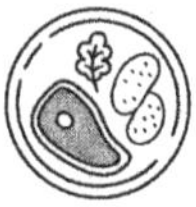 DINNER (FOOD & BEVERAGE)			
BM (HOW MANY BOWEL MOVEMENTS TODAY AND WAS IT HARD OR SOFT, WITH OR WITHOUT STRAINING?			
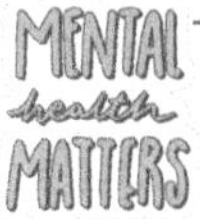	Behavior	Behavior	Behavior

MY FOOD JOURNAL

MEAL	DATE_____	DATE_____	DATE_____
GOOD MORNING BREAKFAST (FOOD & BEVERAGE)			
SNACKS			
LUNCH TIME LUNCH (FOOD & BEVERAGE)			
SNACKS			
DINNER (FOOD & BEVERAGE)			
BM (HOW MANY BOWEL MOVEMENTS TODAY AND WAS IT HARD OR SOFT, WITH OR WITHOUT STRAINING?			
MENTAL health MATTERS	Behavior	Behavior	Behavior

MY FOOD JOURNAL

MEAL	DATE_____	DATE_____	DATE_____
GOOD MORNING BREAKFAST (FOOD & BEVERAGE)			
SNACKS			
LUNCH TIME LUNCH (FOOD & BEVERAGE)			
SNACKS			
DINNER (FOOD & BEVERAGE)			
BM (HOW MANY BOWEL MOVEMENTS TODAY AND WAS IT HARD OR SOFT, WITH OR WITHOUT STRAINING?			
MENTAL health MATTERS	Behavior	Behavior	Behavior

MY FOOD JOURNAL

MEAL	DATE_____	DATE_____	DATE_____
GOOD MORNING BREAKFAST (FOOD & BEVERAGE)			
SNACKS			
LUNCH TIME LUNCH (FOOD & BEVERAGE)			
SNACKS			
DINNER (FOOD & BEVERAGE)			
BM (HOW MANY BOWEL MOVEMENTS TODAY AND WAS IT HARD OR SOFT, WITH OR WITHOUT STRAINING?			
MENTAL health MATTERS	Behavior	Behavior	Behavior

MY FOOD JOURNAL

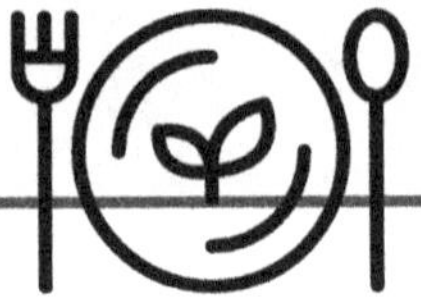

MEAL	DATE_____	DATE_____	DATE_____
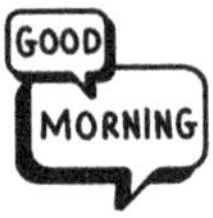 BREAKFAST (FOOD & BEVERAGE)			
SNACKS			
 LUNCH (FOOD & BEVERAGE)			
SNACKS			
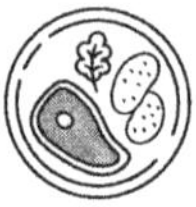 DINNER (FOOD & BEVERAGE)			
BM (HOW MANY BOWEL MOVEMENTS TODAY AND WAS IT HARD OR SOFT, WITH OR WITHOUT STRAINING?			
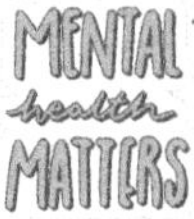	Behavior	Behavior	Behavior

MY FOOD JOURNAL

MEAL	DATE_____	DATE_____	DATE_____
GOOD MORNING BREAKFAST (FOOD & BEVERAGE)			
SNACKS			
LUNCH TIME LUNCH (FOOD & BEVERAGE)			
SNACKS			
DINNER (FOOD & BEVERAGE)			
BM (HOW MANY BOWEL MOVEMENTS TODAY AND WAS IT HARD OR SOFT, WITH OR WITHOUT STRAINING?			
MENTAL health MATTERS	Behavior	Behavior	Behavior

MY FOOD JOURNAL

MEAL	DATE_____	DATE_____	DATE_____
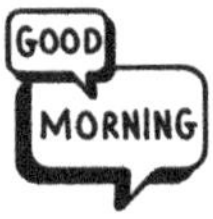 BREAKFAST (FOOD & BEVERAGE)			
SNACKS			
 LUNCH (FOOD & BEVERAGE)			
SNACKS			
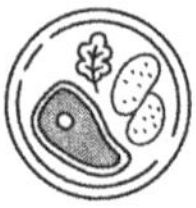 DINNER (FOOD & BEVERAGE)			
BM (HOW MANY BOWEL MOVEMENTS TODAY AND WAS IT HARD OR SOFT, WITH OR WITHOUT STRAINING?			
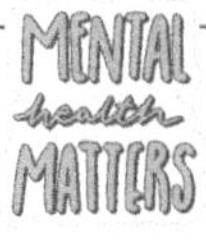	Behavior	Behavior	Behavior

MY FOOD JOURNAL

MEAL	DATE_____	DATE_____	DATE_____
GOOD MORNING BREAKFAST (FOOD & BEVERAGE)			
SNACKS			
LUNCH TIME LUNCH (FOOD & BEVERAGE)			
SNACKS			
DINNER (FOOD & BEVERAGE)			
BM (HOW MANY BOWEL MOVEMENTS TODAY AND WAS IT HARD OR SOFT, WITH OR WITHOUT STRAINING?			
MENTAL health MATTERS	Behavior	Behavior	Behavior

MY FOOD JOURNAL

MEAL	DATE_____	DATE_____	DATE_____
BREAKFAST (FOOD & BEVERAGE)			
SNACKS			
LUNCH (FOOD & BEVERAGE)			
SNACKS			
DINNER (FOOD & BEVERAGE)			
BM (HOW MANY BOWEL MOVEMENTS TODAY AND WAS IT HARD OR SOFT, WITH OR WITHOUT STRAINING?			
	Behavior	Behavior	Behavior

MY FOOD JOURNAL

MEAL	DATE_____	DATE_____	DATE_____
GOOD MORNING BREAKFAST (FOOD & BEVERAGE)			
SNACKS			
LUNCH TIME LUNCH (FOOD & BEVERAGE)			
SNACKS			
DINNER (FOOD & BEVERAGE)			
BM (HOW MANY BOWEL MOVEMENTS TODAY AND WAS IT HARD OR SOFT, WITH OR WITHOUT STRAINING?			
MENTAL health MATTERS	Behavior	Behavior	Behavior

MY FOOD JOURNAL

MEAL	DATE_____	DATE_____	DATE_____
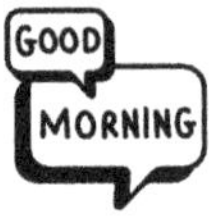 BREAKFAST (FOOD & BEVERAGE)			
SNACKS			
 LUNCH (FOOD & BEVERAGE)			
SNACKS			
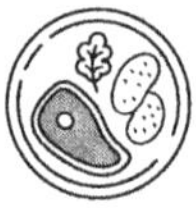 DINNER (FOOD & BEVERAGE)			
BM (HOW MANY BOWEL MOVEMENTS TODAY AND WAS IT HARD OR SOFT, WITH OR WITHOUT STRAINING?			
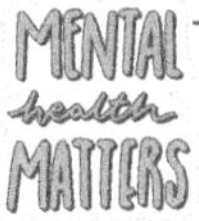	Behavior	Behavior	Behavior

MY FOOD JOURNAL

MEAL	DATE_____	DATE_____	DATE_____
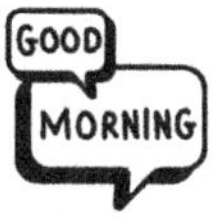 BREAKFAST (FOOD & BEVERAGE)			
SNACKS			
 LUNCH (FOOD & BEVERAGE)			
SNACKS			
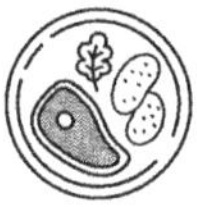 DINNER (FOOD & BEVERAGE)			
BM (HOW MANY BOWEL MOVEMENTS TODAY AND WAS IT HARD OR SOFT, WITH OR WITHOUT STRAINING?			

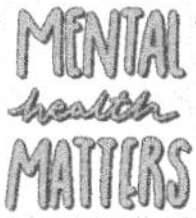

Behavior

Behavior

Behavior

MY FOOD JOURNAL

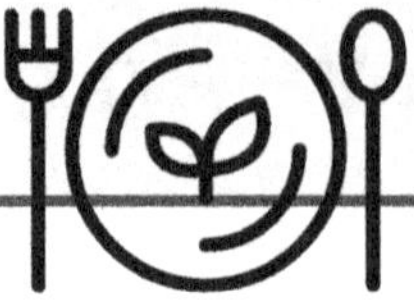

MEAL	DATE_____	DATE_____	DATE_____
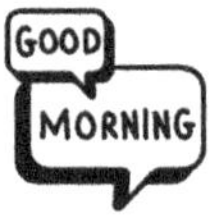 BREAKFAST (FOOD & BEVERAGE)			
SNACKS			
 LUNCH (FOOD & BEVERAGE)			
SNACKS			
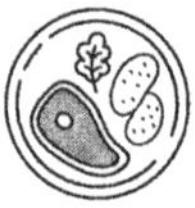 DINNER (FOOD & BEVERAGE)			
BM (HOW MANY BOWEL MOVEMENTS TODAY AND WAS IT HARD OR SOFT, WITH OR WITHOUT STRAINING?			
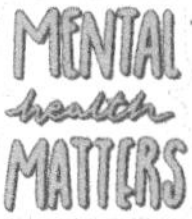	Behavior	Behavior	Behavior

MY FOOD JOURNAL

MEAL	DATE_____	DATE_____	DATE_____
BREAKFAST (FOOD & BEVERAGE)			
SNACKS			
LUNCH (FOOD & BEVERAGE)			
SNACKS			
DINNER (FOOD & BEVERAGE)			
BM (HOW MANY BOWEL MOVEMENTS TODAY AND WAS IT HARD OR SOFT, WITH OR WITHOUT STRAINING?			
	Behavior	Behavior	Behavior

MY FOOD JOURNAL

MEAL	DATE_____	DATE_____	DATE_____
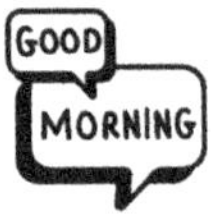 BREAKFAST (FOOD & BEVERAGE)			
SNACKS			
 LUNCH (FOOD & BEVERAGE)			
SNACKS			
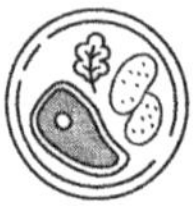 DINNER (FOOD & BEVERAGE)			
BM (HOW MANY BOWEL MOVEMENTS TODAY AND WAS IT HARD OR SOFT, WITH OR WITHOUT STRAINING?			
MENTAL health MATTERS	Behavior	Behavior	Behavior

MY FOOD JOURNAL

MEAL	DATE_____	DATE_____	DATE_____
BREAKFAST (FOOD & BEVERAGE)			
SNACKS			
LUNCH (FOOD & BEVERAGE)			
SNACKS			
DINNER (FOOD & BEVERAGE)			
BM (HOW MANY BOWEL MOVEMENTS TODAY AND WAS IT HARD OR SOFT, WITH OR WITHOUT STRAINING?			
MENTAL health MATTERS	Behavior	Behavior	Behavior

MY FOOD JOURNAL

MEAL	DATE_____	DATE_____	DATE_____
GOOD MORNING BREAKFAST (FOOD & BEVERAGE)			
SNACKS			
LUNCH TIME LUNCH (FOOD & BEVERAGE)			
SNACKS			
DINNER (FOOD & BEVERAGE)			
BM (HOW MANY BOWEL MOVEMENTS TODAY AND WAS IT HARD OR SOFT, WITH OR WITHOUT STRAINING?			
MENTAL health MATTERS	Behavior	Behavior	Behavior

MY FOOD JOURNAL

MEAL	DATE_____	DATE_____	DATE_____
GOOD MORNING BREAKFAST (FOOD & BEVERAGE)			
SNACKS			
LUNCH TIME LUNCH (FOOD & BEVERAGE)			
SNACKS			
DINNER (FOOD & BEVERAGE)			
BM (HOW MANY BOWEL MOVEMENTS TODAY AND WAS IT HARD OR SOFT, WITH OR WITHOUT STRAINING?			
MENTAL health MATTERS	Behavior	Behavior	Behavior

MY FOOD JOURNAL

MEAL	DATE_____	DATE_____	DATE_____
GOOD MORNING BREAKFAST (FOOD & BEVERAGE)			
SNACKS			
LUNCH TIME LUNCH (FOOD & BEVERAGE)			
SNACKS			
DINNER (FOOD & BEVERAGE)			
BM (HOW MANY BOWEL MOVEMENTS TODAY AND WAS IT HARD OR SOFT, WITH OR WITHOUT STRAINING?			
MENTAL health MATTERS	Behavior	Behavior	Behavior

MY FOOD JOURNAL

MEAL	DATE_____	DATE_____	DATE_____
BREAKFAST (FOOD & BEVERAGE)			
SNACKS			
LUNCH (FOOD & BEVERAGE)			
SNACKS			
DINNER (FOOD & BEVERAGE)			
BM (HOW MANY BOWEL MOVEMENTS TODAY AND WAS IT HARD OR SOFT, WITH OR WITHOUT STRAINING?			
	Behavior	Behavior	Behavior

MY FOOD JOURNAL

MEAL	DATE_____	DATE_____	DATE_____
GOOD MORNING BREAKFAST (FOOD & BEVERAGE)			
SNACKS			
LUNCH TIME LUNCH (FOOD & BEVERAGE)			
SNACKS			
DINNER (FOOD & BEVERAGE)			
BM (HOW MANY BOWEL MOVEMENTS TODAY AND WAS IT HARD OR SOFT, WITH OR WITHOUT STRAINING?			
MENTAL health MATTERS	Behavior	Behavior	Behavior

MY FOOD JOURNAL

MEAL	DATE_____	DATE_____	DATE_____
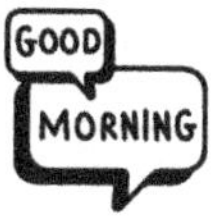 BREAKFAST (FOOD & BEVERAGE)			
SNACKS			
 LUNCH (FOOD & BEVERAGE)			
SNACKS			
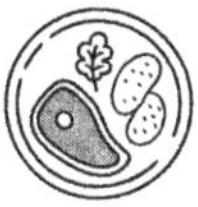 DINNER (FOOD & BEVERAGE)			
BM (HOW MANY BOWEL MOVEMENTS TODAY AND WAS IT HARD OR SOFT, WITH OR WITHOUT STRAINING?			

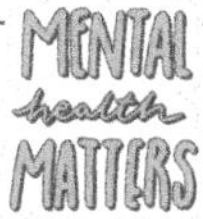

Behavior

Behavior

Behavior

MY FOOD JOURNAL

MEAL	DATE_____	DATE_____	DATE_____
GOOD MORNING BREAKFAST (FOOD & BEVERAGE)			
SNACKS			
LUNCH TIME LUNCH (FOOD & BEVERAGE)			
SNACKS			
DINNER (FOOD & BEVERAGE)			
BM (HOW MANY BOWEL MOVEMENTS TODAY AND WAS IT HARD OR SOFT, WITH OR WITHOUT STRAINING?			
MENTAL health MATTERS	Behavior	Behavior	Behavior

MY FOOD JOURNAL

MEAL	DATE_____	DATE_____	DATE_____
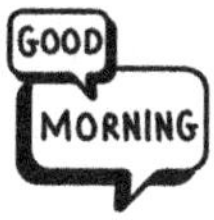 BREAKFAST (FOOD & BEVERAGE)			
SNACKS			
 LUNCH (FOOD & BEVERAGE)			
SNACKS			
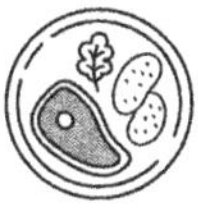 DINNER (FOOD & BEVERAGE)			
BM (HOW MANY BOWEL MOVEMENTS TODAY AND WAS IT HARD OR SOFT, WITH OR WITHOUT STRAINING?			

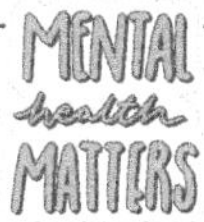

Behavior

Behavior

Behavior

MY FOOD JOURNAL

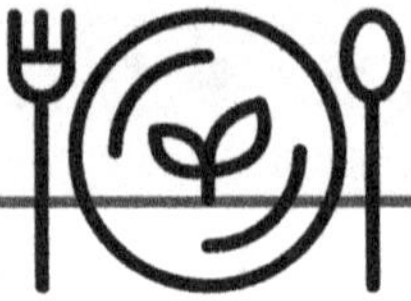

MEAL	DATE_____	DATE_____	DATE_____
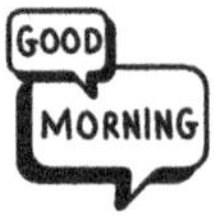 BREAKFAST (FOOD & BEVERAGE)			
SNACKS			
 LUNCH (FOOD & BEVERAGE)			
SNACKS			
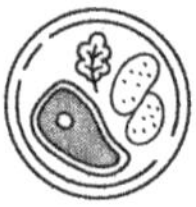 DINNER (FOOD & BEVERAGE)			
BM (HOW MANY BOWEL MOVEMENTS TODAY AND WAS IT HARD OR SOFT, WITH OR WITHOUT STRAINING?			

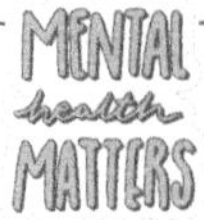

Behavior

Behavior

Behavior

MY FOOD JOURNAL

MEAL	DATE_____	DATE_____	DATE_____
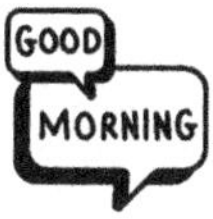 BREAKFAST (FOOD & BEVERAGE)			
SNACKS			
 LUNCH (FOOD & BEVERAGE)			
SNACKS			
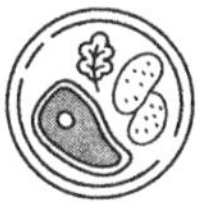 DINNER (FOOD & BEVERAGE)			
BM (HOW MANY BOWEL MOVEMENTS TODAY AND WAS IT HARD OR SOFT, WITH OR WITHOUT STRAINING?			

MENTAL health MATTERS

Behavior

Behavior

Behavior

MY FOOD JOURNAL

MEAL	DATE_____	DATE_____	DATE_____
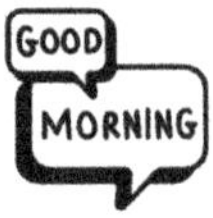 BREAKFAST (FOOD & BEVERAGE)			
SNACKS			
 LUNCH (FOOD & BEVERAGE)			
SNACKS			
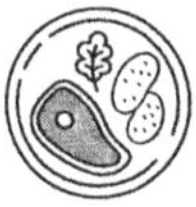 DINNER (FOOD & BEVERAGE)			
BM (HOW MANY BOWEL MOVEMENTS TODAY AND WAS IT HARD OR SOFT, WITH OR WITHOUT STRAINING?			
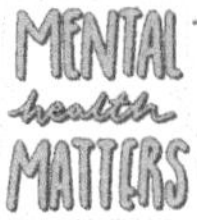	Behavior	Behavior	Behavior

MY FOOD JOURNAL

MEAL	DATE_____	DATE_____	DATE_____
BREAKFAST (FOOD & BEVERAGE)			
SNACKS			
LUNCH (FOOD & BEVERAGE)			
SNACKS			
DINNER (FOOD & BEVERAGE)			
BM (HOW MANY BOWEL MOVEMENTS TODAY AND WAS IT HARD OR SOFT, WITH OR WITHOUT STRAINING?			
	Behavior	Behavior	Behavior

MY FOOD JOURNAL

MEAL	DATE_____	DATE_____	DATE_____
GOOD MORNING BREAKFAST (FOOD & BEVERAGE)			
SNACKS			
LUNCH TIME LUNCH (FOOD & BEVERAGE)			
SNACKS			
DINNER (FOOD & BEVERAGE)			
BM (HOW MANY BOWEL MOVEMENTS TODAY AND WAS IT HARD OR SOFT, WITH OR WITHOUT STRAINING?			
MENTAL health MATTERS	Behavior	Behavior	Behavior

MY FOOD JOURNAL

MEAL	DATE_____	DATE_____	DATE_____
GOOD MORNING BREAKFAST (FOOD & BEVERAGE)			
SNACKS			
LUNCH TIME LUNCH (FOOD & BEVERAGE)			
SNACKS			
DINNER (FOOD & BEVERAGE)			
BM (HOW MANY BOWEL MOVEMENTS TODAY AND WAS IT HARD OR SOFT, WITH OR WITHOUT STRAINING?			

MENTAL health MATTERS

Behavior	Behavior	Behavior

MY FOOD JOURNAL

MEAL	DATE_____	DATE_____	DATE_____
BREAKFAST (FOOD & BEVERAGE)			
SNACKS			
LUNCH (FOOD & BEVERAGE)			
SNACKS			
DINNER (FOOD & BEVERAGE)			
BM (HOW MANY BOWEL MOVEMENTS TODAY AND WAS IT HARD OR SOFT, WITH OR WITHOUT STRAINING?			
	Behavior	Behavior	Behavior

MY FOOD JOURNAL

MEAL	DATE_____	DATE_____	DATE_____
GOOD MORNING BREAKFAST (FOOD & BEVERAGE)			
SNACKS			
LUNCH TIME LUNCH (FOOD & BEVERAGE)			
SNACKS			
DINNER (FOOD & BEVERAGE)			
BM (HOW MANY BOWEL MOVEMENTS TODAY AND WAS IT HARD OR SOFT, WITH OR WITHOUT STRAINING?			
MENTAL health MATTERS	Behavior	Behavior	Behavior

MY FOOD JOURNAL

MEAL	DATE_____	DATE_____	DATE_____
GOOD MORNING BREAKFAST (FOOD & BEVERAGE)			
SNACKS			
LUNCH TIME LUNCH (FOOD & BEVERAGE)			
SNACKS			
DINNER (FOOD & BEVERAGE)			
BM (HOW MANY BOWEL MOVEMENTS TODAY AND WAS IT HARD OR SOFT, WITH OR WITHOUT STRAINING?			
MENTAL health MATTERS	Behavior	Behavior	Behavior

MY FOOD JOURNAL

MEAL	DATE_____	DATE_____	DATE_____
GOOD MORNING BREAKFAST (FOOD & BEVERAGE)			
SNACKS			
LUNCH TIME LUNCH (FOOD & BEVERAGE)			
SNACKS			
DINNER (FOOD & BEVERAGE)			
BM (HOW MANY BOWEL MOVEMENTS TODAY AND WAS IT HARD OR SOFT, WITH OR WITHOUT STRAINING?			
MENTAL health MATTERS	Behavior	Behavior	Behavior

MY FOOD JOURNAL

MEAL	DATE_____	DATE_____	DATE_____
GOOD MORNING BREAKFAST (FOOD & BEVERAGE)			
SNACKS			
LUNCH TIME LUNCH (FOOD & BEVERAGE)			
SNACKS			
DINNER (FOOD & BEVERAGE)			
BM (HOW MANY BOWEL MOVEMENTS TODAY AND WAS IT HARD OR SOFT, WITH OR WITHOUT STRAINING?			
MENTAL health MATTERS	Behavior	Behavior	Behavior

MY FOOD JOURNAL

MEAL	DATE_____	DATE_____	DATE_____
GOOD MORNING BREAKFAST (FOOD & BEVERAGE)			
SNACKS			
LUNCH TIME LUNCH (FOOD & BEVERAGE)			
SNACKS			
DINNER (FOOD & BEVERAGE)			
BM (HOW MANY BOWEL MOVEMENTS TODAY AND WAS IT HARD OR SOFT, WITH OR WITHOUT STRAINING?			
MENTAL health MATTERS	Behavior	Behavior	Behavior

MY FOOD JOURNAL

MEAL	DATE_____	DATE_____	DATE_____
GOOD MORNING BREAKFAST (FOOD & BEVERAGE)			
SNACKS			
LUNCH TIME LUNCH (FOOD & BEVERAGE)			
SNACKS			
DINNER (FOOD & BEVERAGE)			
BM (HOW MANY BOWEL MOVEMENTS TODAY AND WAS IT HARD OR SOFT, WITH OR WITHOUT STRAINING?			
MENTAL health MATTERS	Behavior	Behavior	Behavior

MY FOOD JOURNAL

MEAL	DATE_____	DATE_____	DATE_____
GOOD MORNING BREAKFAST (FOOD & BEVERAGE)			
SNACKS			
LUNCH TIME LUNCH (FOOD & BEVERAGE)			
SNACKS			
DINNER (FOOD & BEVERAGE)			
BM (HOW MANY BOWEL MOVEMENTS TODAY AND WAS IT HARD OR SOFT, WITH OR WITHOUT STRAINING?			
MENTAL health MATTERS	Behavior	Behavior	Behavior

MY FOOD JOURNAL

MEAL	DATE_____	DATE_____	DATE_____
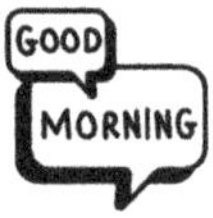 BREAKFAST (FOOD & BEVERAGE)			
SNACKS			
 LUNCH (FOOD & BEVERAGE)			
SNACKS			
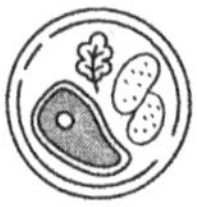 DINNER (FOOD & BEVERAGE)			
BM (HOW MANY BOWEL MOVEMENTS TODAY AND WAS IT HARD OR SOFT, WITH OR WITHOUT STRAINING?			
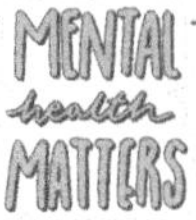	Behavior	Behavior	Behavior

MY FOOD JOURNAL

MEAL	DATE_____	DATE_____	DATE_____
GOOD MORNING BREAKFAST (FOOD & BEVERAGE)			
SNACKS			
LUNCH TIME LUNCH (FOOD & BEVERAGE)			
SNACKS			
DINNER (FOOD & BEVERAGE)			
BM (HOW MANY BOWEL MOVEMENTS TODAY AND WAS IT HARD OR SOFT, WITH OR WITHOUT STRAINING?			
MENTAL health MATTERS	Behavior	Behavior	Behavior

MY FOOD JOURNAL

MEAL	DATE_____	DATE_____	DATE_____
BREAKFAST (FOOD & BEVERAGE)			
SNACKS			
LUNCH (FOOD & BEVERAGE)			
SNACKS			
DINNER (FOOD & BEVERAGE)			
BM (HOW MANY BOWEL MOVEMENTS TODAY AND WAS IT HARD OR SOFT, WITH OR WITHOUT STRAINING?			
	Behavior	Behavior	Behavior

MY FOOD JOURNAL

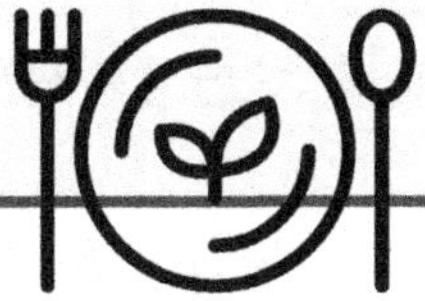

MEAL	DATE_____	DATE_____	DATE_____
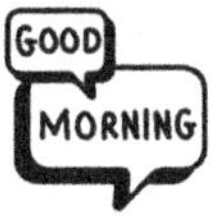 BREAKFAST (FOOD & BEVERAGE)			
SNACKS			
 LUNCH (FOOD & BEVERAGE)			
SNACKS			
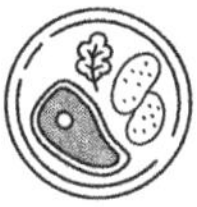 DINNER (FOOD & BEVERAGE)			
BM (HOW MANY BOWEL MOVEMENTS TODAY AND WAS IT HARD OR SOFT, WITH OR WITHOUT STRAINING?			

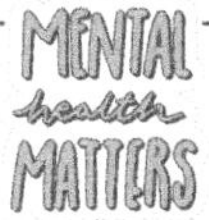

Behavior	Behavior	Behavior

MY FOOD JOURNAL

MEAL	DATE_____	DATE_____	DATE_____
BREAKFAST (FOOD & BEVERAGE)			
SNACKS			
LUNCH (FOOD & BEVERAGE)			
SNACKS			
DINNER (FOOD & BEVERAGE)			
BM (HOW MANY BOWEL MOVEMENTS TODAY AND WAS IT HARD OR SOFT, WITH OR WITHOUT STRAINING?			
	Behavior	Behavior	Behavior

MY FOOD JOURNAL

MEAL	DATE_____	DATE_____	DATE_____
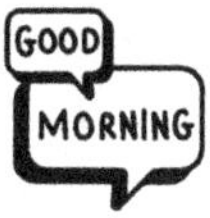 BREAKFAST (FOOD & BEVERAGE)			
SNACKS			
 LUNCH (FOOD & BEVERAGE)			
SNACKS			
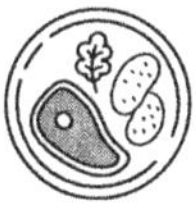 DINNER (FOOD & BEVERAGE)			
BM (HOW MANY BOWEL MOVEMENTS TODAY AND WAS IT HARD OR SOFT, WITH OR WITHOUT STRAINING?			

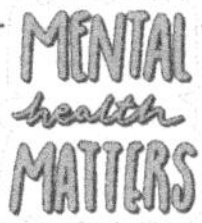

Behavior | Behavior | Behavior

MY FOOD JOURNAL

MEAL	DATE_____	DATE_____	DATE_____
GOOD MORNING BREAKFAST (FOOD & BEVERAGE)			
SNACKS			
LUNCH TIME LUNCH (FOOD & BEVERAGE)			
SNACKS			
DINNER (FOOD & BEVERAGE)			
BM (HOW MANY BOWEL MOVEMENTS TODAY AND WAS IT HARD OR SOFT, WITH OR WITHOUT STRAINING?			
MENTAL health MATTERS	Behavior	Behavior	Behavior

MY FOOD JOURNAL

MEAL	DATE_____	DATE_____	DATE_____
BREAKFAST (FOOD & BEVERAGE)			
SNACKS			
LUNCH (FOOD & BEVERAGE)			
SNACKS			
DINNER (FOOD & BEVERAGE)			
BM (HOW MANY BOWEL MOVEMENTS TODAY AND WAS IT HARD OR SOFT, WITH OR WITHOUT STRAINING?			

Behavior	Behavior	Behavior

MY FOOD JOURNAL

MEAL	DATE_____	DATE_____	DATE_____
GOOD MORNING BREAKFAST (FOOD & BEVERAGE)			
SNACKS			
LUNCH TIME LUNCH (FOOD & BEVERAGE)			
SNACKS			
DINNER (FOOD & BEVERAGE)			
BM (HOW MANY BOWEL MOVEMENTS TODAY AND WAS IT HARD OR SOFT, WITH OR WITHOUT STRAINING?			
MENTAL health MATTERS	Behavior	Behavior	Behavior

MY FOOD JOURNAL

MEAL	DATE_____	DATE_____	DATE_____
GOOD MORNING BREAKFAST (FOOD & BEVERAGE)			
SNACKS			
LUNCH TIME LUNCH (FOOD & BEVERAGE)			
SNACKS			
DINNER (FOOD & BEVERAGE)			
BM (HOW MANY BOWEL MOVEMENTS TODAY AND WAS IT HARD OR SOFT, WITH OR WITHOUT STRAINING?			

MENTAL health MATTERS

Behavior	Behavior	Behavior

MY FOOD JOURNAL

MEAL	DATE_____	DATE_____	DATE_____
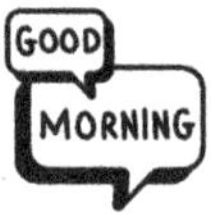 BREAKFAST (FOOD & BEVERAGE)			
SNACKS			
 LUNCH (FOOD & BEVERAGE)			
SNACKS			
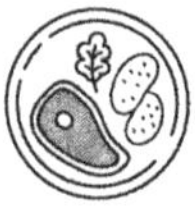 DINNER (FOOD & BEVERAGE)			
BM (HOW MANY BOWEL MOVEMENTS TODAY AND WAS IT HARD OR SOFT, WITH OR WITHOUT STRAINING?			
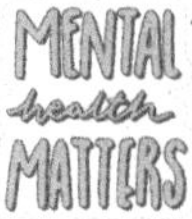	Behavior	Behavior	Behavior

MY FOOD JOURNAL

MEAL	DATE_____	DATE_____	DATE_____
GOOD MORNING BREAKFAST (FOOD & BEVERAGE)			
SNACKS			
LUNCH TIME LUNCH (FOOD & BEVERAGE)			
SNACKS			
DINNER (FOOD & BEVERAGE)			
BM (HOW MANY BOWEL MOVEMENTS TODAY AND WAS IT HARD OR SOFT, WITH OR WITHOUT STRAINING?			

MENTAL health MATTERS

Behavior | Behavior | Behavior

MY FOOD JOURNAL

MEAL	DATE_____	DATE_____	DATE_____
BREAKFAST (FOOD & BEVERAGE)			
SNACKS			
LUNCH (FOOD & BEVERAGE)			
SNACKS			
DINNER (FOOD & BEVERAGE)			
BM (HOW MANY BOWEL MOVEMENTS TODAY AND WAS IT HARD OR SOFT, WITH OR WITHOUT STRAINING?			

Behavior

Behavior

Behavior

MY FOOD JOURNAL

MEAL	DATE_____	DATE_____	DATE_____
GOOD MORNING BREAKFAST (FOOD & BEVERAGE)			
SNACKS			
LUNCH TIME LUNCH (FOOD & BEVERAGE)			
SNACKS			
DINNER (FOOD & BEVERAGE)			
BM (HOW MANY BOWEL MOVEMENTS TODAY AND WAS IT HARD OR SOFT, WITH OR WITHOUT STRAINING?			

MENTAL health MATTERS

	Behavior	Behavior	Behavior

MY FOOD JOURNAL

MEAL	DATE_____	DATE_____	DATE_____
GOOD MORNING BREAKFAST (FOOD & BEVERAGE)			
SNACKS			
LUNCH TIME LUNCH (FOOD & BEVERAGE)			
SNACKS			
DINNER (FOOD & BEVERAGE)			
BM (HOW MANY BOWEL MOVEMENTS TODAY AND WAS IT HARD OR SOFT, WITH OR WITHOUT STRAINING?			
MENTAL health MATTERS	Behavior	Behavior	Behavior

MY FOOD JOURNAL

MEAL	DATE_____	DATE_____	DATE_____
GOOD MORNING BREAKFAST (FOOD & BEVERAGE)			
SNACKS			
LUNCH TIME LUNCH (FOOD & BEVERAGE)			
SNACKS			
DINNER (FOOD & BEVERAGE)			
BM (HOW MANY BOWEL MOVEMENTS TODAY AND WAS IT HARD OR SOFT, WITH OR WITHOUT STRAINING?			
MENTAL health MATTERS	Behavior	Behavior	Behavior

MY FOOD JOURNAL

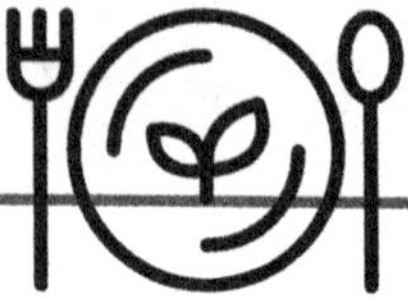

MEAL	DATE_____	DATE_____	DATE_____
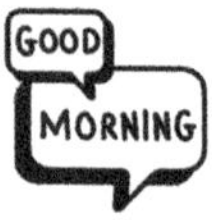 BREAKFAST (FOOD & BEVERAGE)			
SNACKS			
 LUNCH (FOOD & BEVERAGE)			
SNACKS			
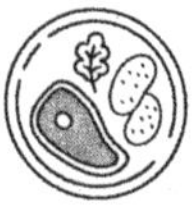 DINNER (FOOD & BEVERAGE)			
BM (HOW MANY BOWEL MOVEMENTS TODAY AND WAS IT HARD OR SOFT, WITH OR WITHOUT STRAINING?			
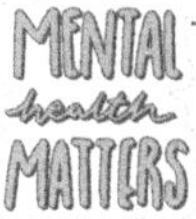	Behavior	Behavior	Behavior

MY FOOD JOURNAL

MEAL	DATE_____	DATE_____	DATE_____
GOOD MORNING BREAKFAST (FOOD & BEVERAGE)			
SNACKS			
LUNCH TIME LUNCH (FOOD & BEVERAGE)			
SNACKS			
DINNER (FOOD & BEVERAGE)			
BM (HOW MANY BOWEL MOVEMENTS TODAY AND WAS IT HARD OR SOFT, WITH OR WITHOUT STRAINING?			

MENTAL health MATTERS

Behavior

Behavior

Behavior

MY FOOD JOURNAL

MEAL	DATE_____	DATE_____	DATE_____
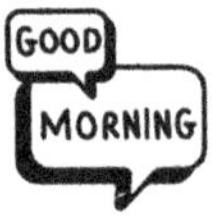 BREAKFAST (FOOD & BEVERAGE)			
SNACKS			
 LUNCH (FOOD & BEVERAGE)			
SNACKS			
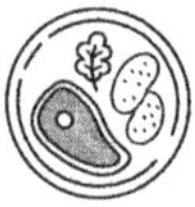 DINNER (FOOD & BEVERAGE)			
BM (HOW MANY BOWEL MOVEMENTS TODAY AND WAS IT HARD OR SOFT, WITH OR WITHOUT STRAINING?			
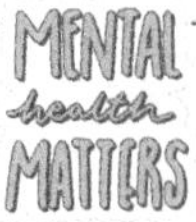	Behavior	Behavior	Behavior

Made in the USA
Monee, IL
04 November 2026

67387472R10066